SAMMiE & SAX
in the Land of Quinoa

Sheila Kemper Dietrich is the Founder and CEO of Livliga—a brand of healthy, artist-designed dinnerware products to help people and families live healthier lives.

Timothy Foss is the Chief Creative Officer of Livliga.

VisualQs, LLC, Boulder 80308

www.livligahome.com

©2013 by VisualQs, LLC

Printed in China.

20 19 18 17 16 15 14 13   1 2 3 4 5 6

ISBN-10: 0989014908 (Hardcover)

ISBN-13: 978-0-9890149-0-8 (Hardcover)

Library of Congress Control Number: 2013933220

This paper meets the requirements of
ISO 9706 (Permanence of Paper)

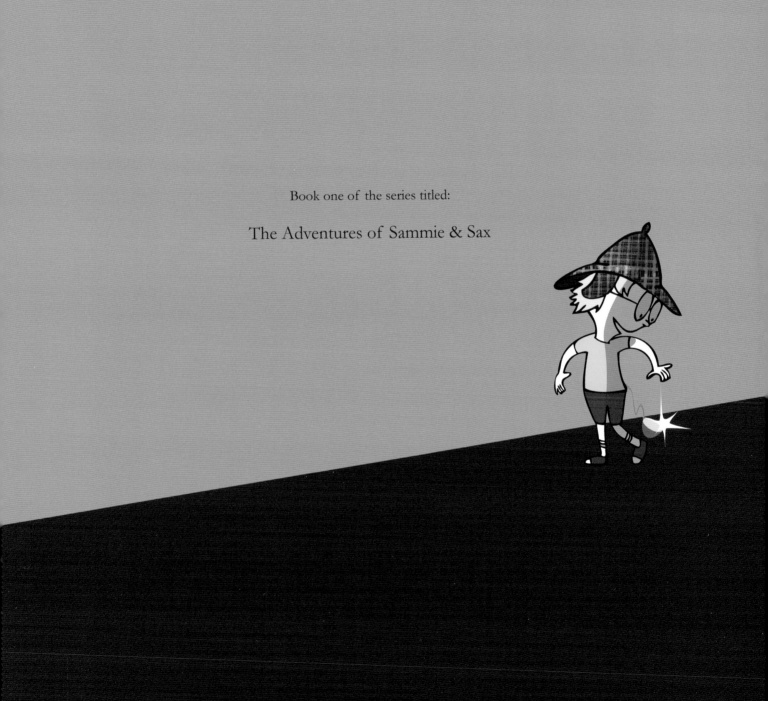

Book one of the series titled:

The Adventures of Sammie & Sax

A Note of Gratitude and Thanks

Often acknowledgments end with thanking the family. I wanted to start by thanking mine. I am one lucky woman to have an amazing husband who not only encouraged me but also rearranged his life to help support me in fulfilling my dream of making this book and the overall children's line of Livliga come to life. I also want to thank my three terrific children. Each of them has acted as cheerleader and counselor to me at critical points in the creative process of this book. Fate played an important part in bringing Livliga, Sammie and Sax, and this book to life. Being introduced to the very talented Tim Foss made the caliber and content of these creations both fun and fabulous. It has made the adventure that much more rewarding and fun.

How truly blessed I am to have such great friends of many professions and talents who were willing to take on a collaboration and tasks like editing and scrutinizing the pages of this book because they believed in the project and believed it was possible to make it come to life. Specific thanks to these great friends—Enid Dodson, Margo Humenczuk, Michelle Bolton King and Kit Nathan Smith.

Sheila Kemper Dietrich

I dedicate this book to Dana Elkun and Eli Jupiter, my new family, for giving me the reason to finally grow up. I thank my mother, father, and brother for letting me take my time at it. I thank Sheila and Walt for the gift of telling a story that can help all families love good, healthy food.

Tim Foss

Foreword

Dear Fellow Parents,

As a mother, I want the very best for my daughter. I know that it is my job to teach her how to be the best person she can be, both inside and out. I am afraid for her because obesity runs in my family, and she has Down syndrome, which causes a slow metabolism at a very early age. Children need to be taught how to eat well, so we have tried to model healthy eating choices for Emma ever since she was a baby.

There is now a wonderful tool to help teach healthy eating choices to young children. Through its engaging story and beautiful illustrations, Sheila Dietrich and Tim Foss have brought to life how fun and delicious it can be to eat a balanced meal. As an educator, I see this book as an invaluable resource for parents, educators, child-care providers, and medical professionals who want to teach children how to lead healthy lifestyles at an early age and battle the increasing cases of childhood obesity. As a mother, I see this book as an enchanting story to read with my daughter.

Enid Dodson
National Consultant and School Designer, Expeditionary Learning

Introduction

Dear Parent, Grandparent or Child Advocate,

Having helped the Dietrich family with nutrition while their children were young, I am pleased to introduce you to Sheila Kemper Dietrich's new book and to Sammie and Sax in their adventure to search for a balanced meal.

Before super-sized restaurant meals, highly processed, sweetened, or fried "snacks," and sweetened beverages were regularly consumed by children, most children were naturally at a healthy weight and in good health.

As a registered dietitian and board certified specialist in pediatric nutrition, I can't stress enough how essential developing good eating habits early in childhood is for all children for lifelong health. Children who are exposed to a variety of healthy foods served in age appropriate serving sizes learn healthy eating habits that will help them be healthy lifelong.

Most children love eating a variety of foods and enjoy them even more when they participate in growing, selecting, or preparing foods. For those who are more timid eaters, introducing foods with a great story and a spirit of adventure can unlock the child's natural curiosity and make trying new foods more fun. Help your child learn to enjoy good eating habits with this exciting adventure and serve up some appetizing, healthy food on the children's line of Livliga dinnerware.

Every kid loves an adventure, and with the story of Sammie and Sax, Sheila Kemper Dietrich introduces healthy eating in a way that appeals to a child's adventurous spirit. A trip to a farmers' market is always fun, and the variety of healthy fruit, vegetables, grains and often even meat and dairy items is broad enough for every child to find some appealing new food to try. Learning to select, prepare, and enjoy healthy food is a great family experience all children should have. Livliga dinnerware provides a fun tool to guide your child to healthy eating. Join Sammie and Sax to see what fun, healthy eating can be.

Margo Murray Humenczuk, MA, MBA, RD, CSP, LD

SAMMiE & SAX in the Land of Quinoa

the search for a balanced meal

Sheila Kemper Dietrich

illustrated by
Timothy Foss

VisualQs, LLC, Boulder, Colorado

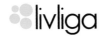

livliga

"Good morning, Mama!" Sammie sings as she skips into the kitchen. "Breakfast looks yummy! What's for dinner? Can we have potato chips and dip?"

"Or ice cream cones with cookies!" adds little brother, Sax, as he lifts his head from his book.

Mama laughs, "Well, I know you two love those foods, but we'll need to plan a more balanced meal. Could you help me make a grocery list?"

"Sure! But what's a balanced meal?" Sammie says through a bite of toast. Their mother is about to reply, when SUDDENLY...

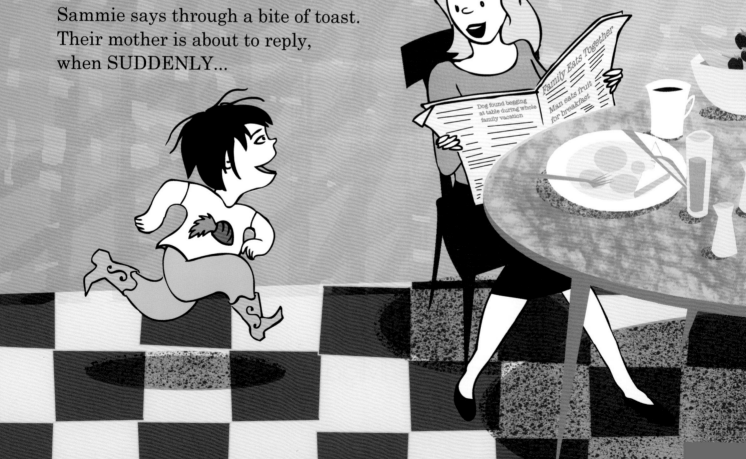

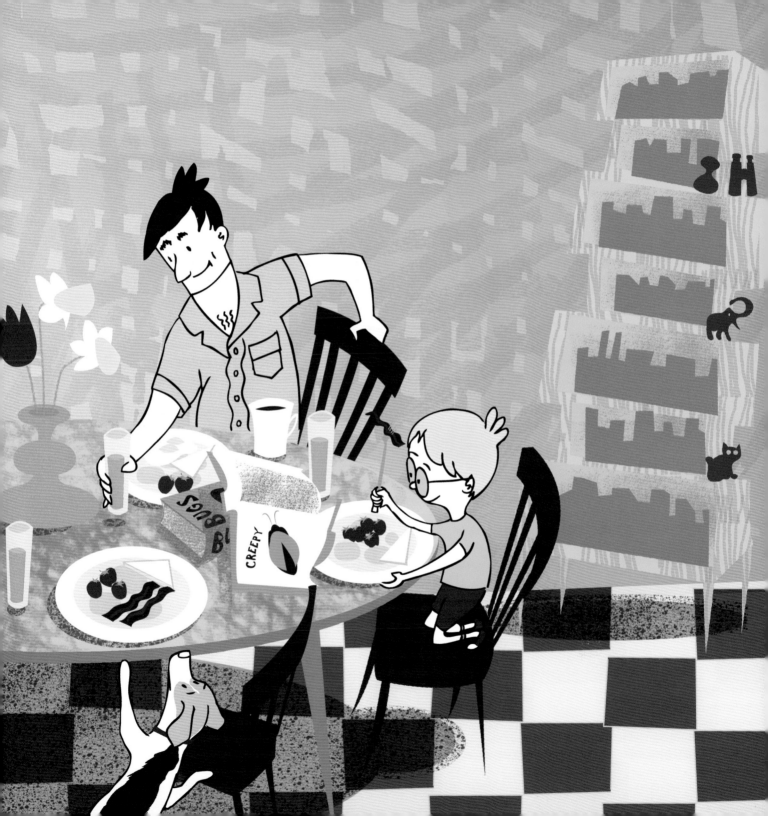

"ACHOO!!"

Sax sneezes then pulls his well-worn cap onto his head. "Excuse me,
my *curiosity cap* makes me sneeze. But NEVER FEAR! Now I'm
READY TO THINK!"

"WROOF! WROOF!" barks Rhubarb, as he chomps a morsel of bacon.

Sammie swallows her bite and adds,
"But where do we start?"

"Why not look in our
cookbooks?" Mama
answers, sipping
her coffee.

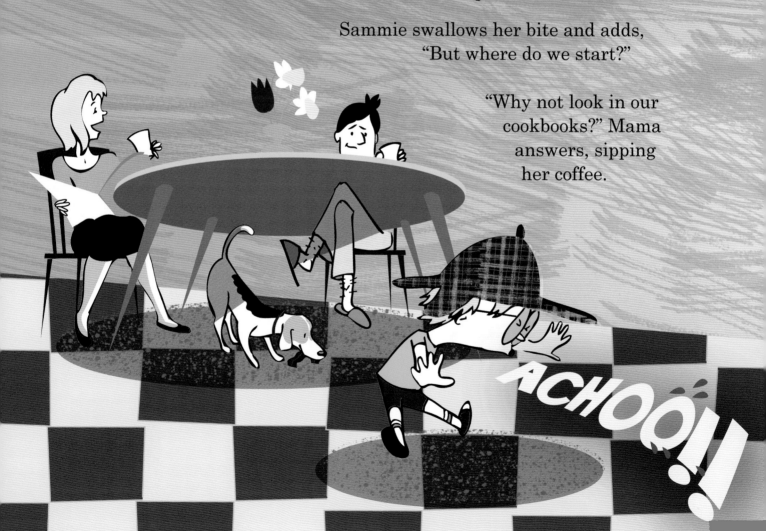

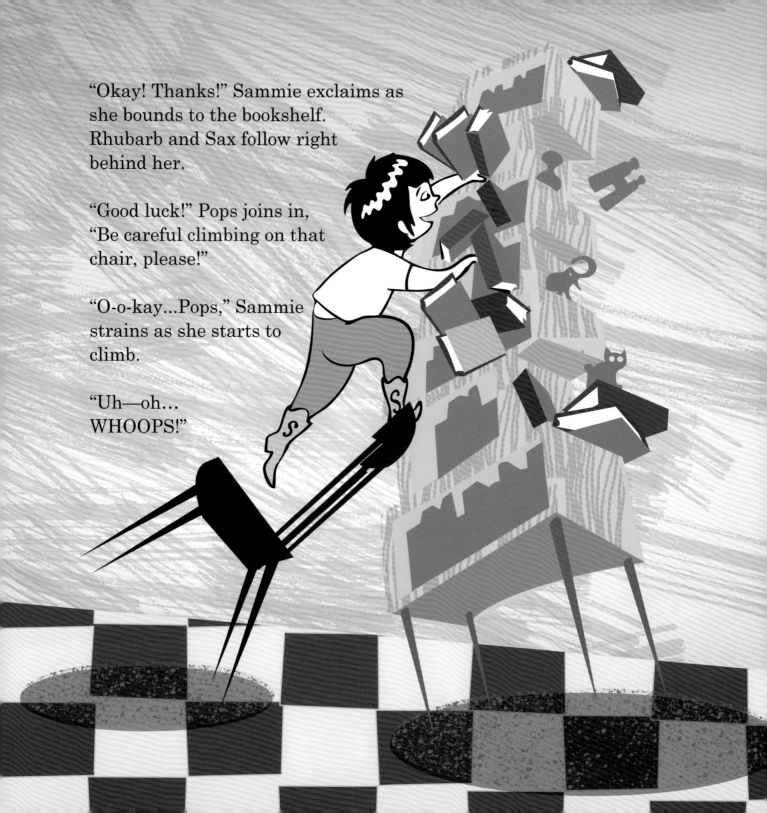

"Okay! Thanks!" Sammie exclaims as she bounds to the bookshelf. Rhubarb and Sax follow right behind her.

"Good luck!" Pops joins in, "Be careful climbing on that chair, please!"

"O-o-kay...Pops," Sammie strains as she starts to climb.

"Uh—oh... WHOOPS!"

CRASH!!!!

"WROOF!" barks Rhubarb.

"OUCH!" yells Sax. "So—rry," Sammie apologizes then looks at the mess of books around her.

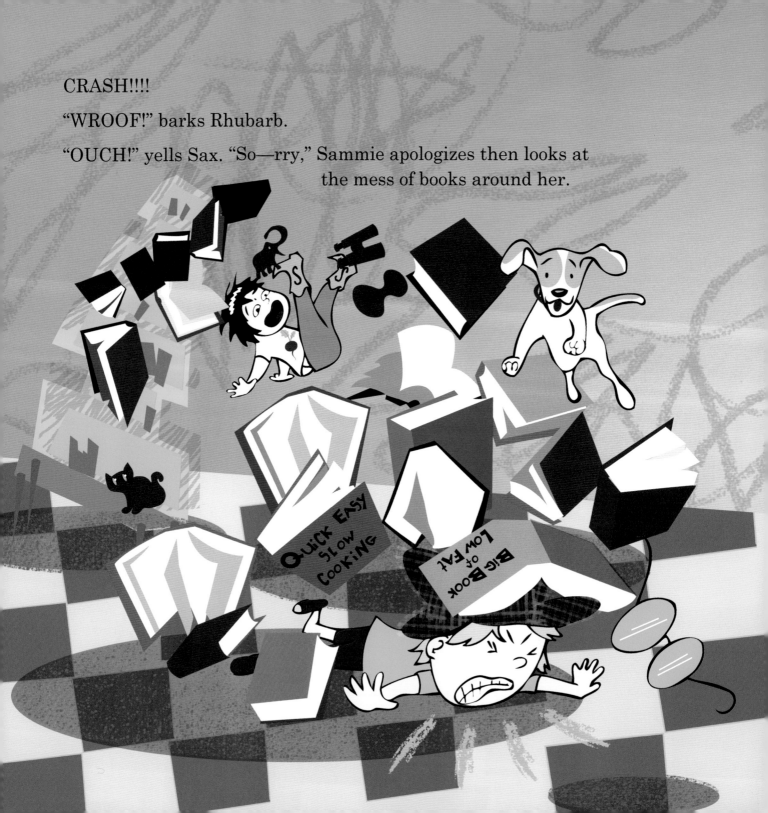

"Umpff," groans Sax as he straightens his glasses.

"Look in this book!" He points, "Here's a plate full of vegetables and fish and something that looks like a sweet potato."

"Sweet potatoes, yum! My favorite!" Sammie says as she plops down next to the stack of books by her brother. "How do we know if all that food makes a balanced meal?"

"Good question!" Sax answers.

"Sax, did you say 'GOOD QUESTION!'?" Sammie asks, then gives her brother a big smile and a wink.

Sax flashes an even bigger smile back and says, "I sure did, Sammie!" and even before Rhubarb can bark, they race to the kitchen drawer shouting,

"Time for a *SPOON ZOOM!*"

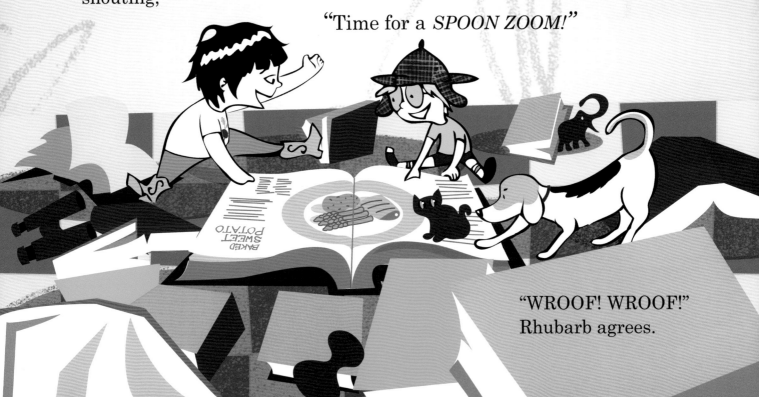

"WROOF! WROOF!"
Rhubarb agrees.

"The magic LivSpoon," Sammie whispers to her brother as they admire it together.

"Look how it sparkles," says Sax. "It always looks ready for an adventure!"

Sax grabs the LivSpoon firmly.

Sammie says, "Climb on board, little brother!" and Sax jumps up on Sammie's back.

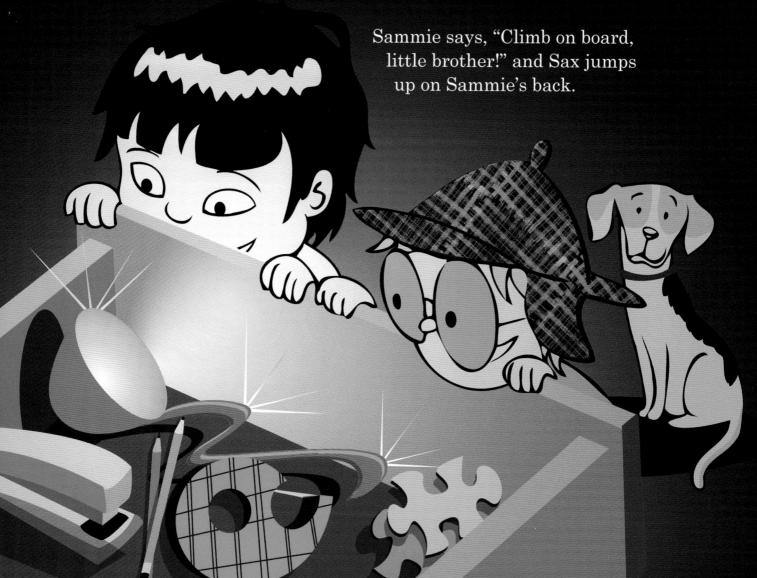

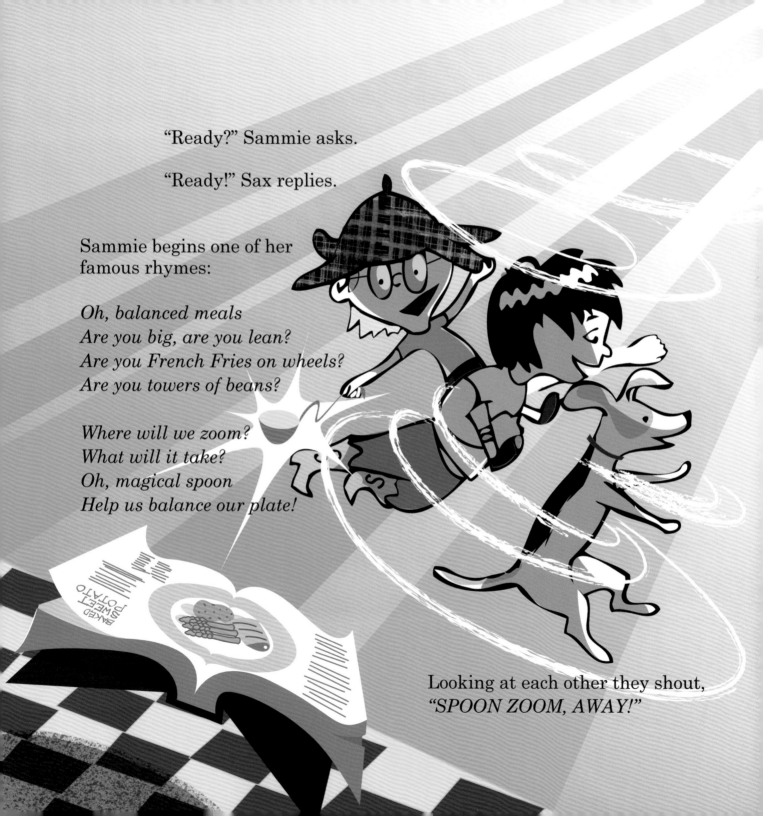

"Ready?" Sammie asks.

"Ready!" Sax replies.

Sammie begins one of her
famous rhymes:

Oh, balanced meals
Are you big, are you lean?
Are you French Fries on wheels?
Are you towers of beans?

Where will we zoom?
What will it take?
Oh, magical spoon
Help us balance our plate!

Looking at each other they shout,
"SPOON ZOOM, AWAY!"

"Sax! Look at all these foods! I mean puzzle pieces! I mean food puzzles! Or people foods! WHATEVER! Just look! They all talk and move! What an awesome magical land!"

"ACHOO!!" Sax sneezes while trying to adjust his curiosity cap. "Aha!" he says, with clear thinking, "It appears we're in a magical land of talking puzzle people foods!"

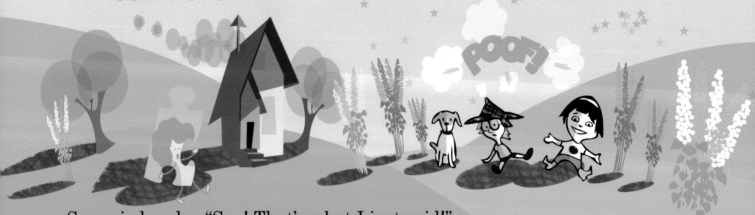

Sammie laughs, "Sax! That's what I just said!"

"Welcome to the Land of Quinoa, children," waves the carrot puzzle piece who is walking by on her way to town.

"Keen who?!" Sammie wonders aloud.

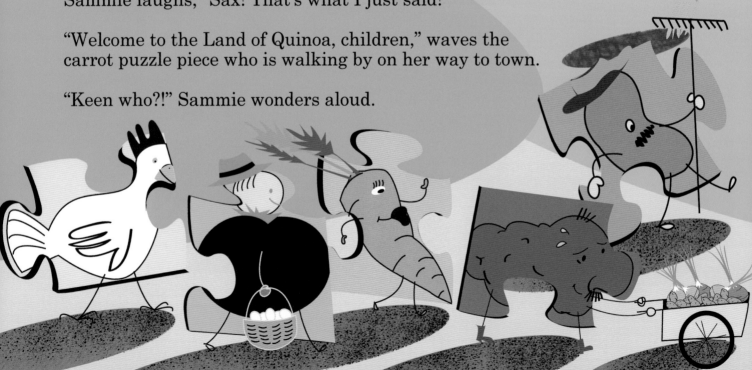

"Keen-wah," answers a large broccoli puzzle piece. "It's a tasty little grain that pops when you chew it. It grows all around here. I'm Ms. Broccoli, nice to meet you. What brings you to my front yard?"

"I'm Sammie, and this is my brother, Sax," Sammie replies.

"We are here on a mission to balance meals!" Sax chimes in loudly.

Ms. Broccoli laughs kindly saying, "Ah, learning about balanced meals, are you?"

"Yes!" Sammie blurts out, "that's it! You sure look dee—licious! Are you a balanced meal?"

"Well, I am gorgeous with lovely green florets," Ms. Broccoli explains proudly. "And I'm absolutely packed full of calcium—just like milk—to help your bones grow strong. But..." she sighs, "I'm not a balanced meal. Now I must tend to my flowers, children, and get them to the market!"

"Okay, thanks!" waves Sammie, following Sax and Rhubarb down the road.

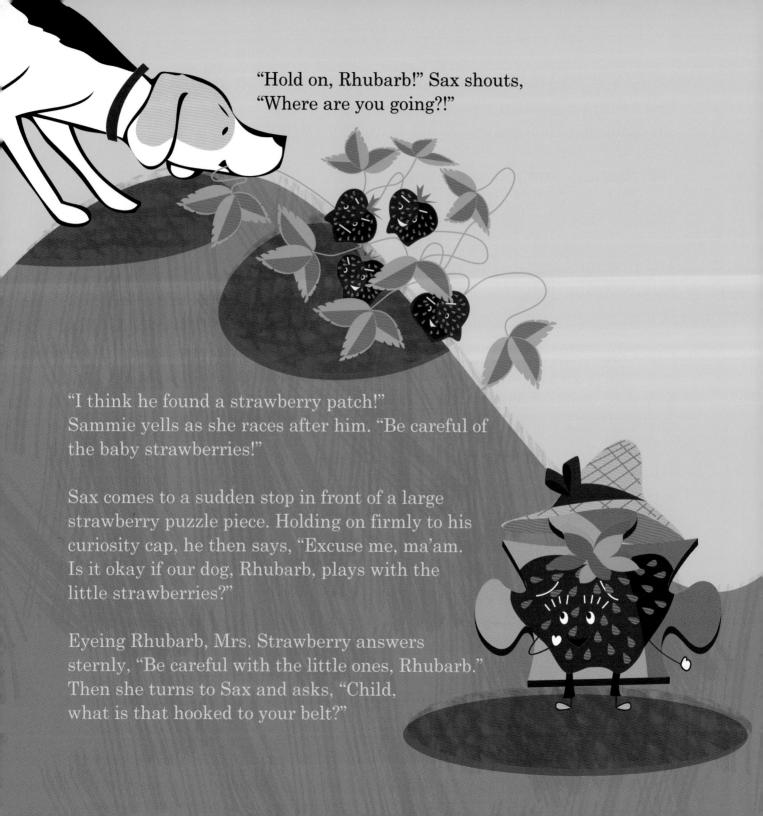

"Hold on, Rhubarb!" Sax shouts,
"Where are you going?!"

"I think he found a strawberry patch!"
Sammie yells as she races after him. "Be careful of
the baby strawberries!"

Sax comes to a sudden stop in front of a large
strawberry puzzle piece. Holding on firmly to his
curiosity cap, he then says, "Excuse me, ma'am.
Is it okay if our dog, Rhubarb, plays with the
little strawberries?"

Eyeing Rhubarb, Mrs. Strawberry answers
sternly, "Be careful with the little ones, Rhubarb."
Then she turns to Sax and asks, "Child,
what is that hooked to your belt?"

Sax, looking surprised, answers, "Oh, that is our LivSpoon! It delivered us here on our mission to discover balanced meals! Are you one?"

"Well, I am bright red and polka-dotted with charming seeds. Cooks just adore me because of the way I make any meal look beautiful. Doctors know that I help people fight diseases, and I even won an award for being one of the most heart-healthy fruits! But no matter how famous I might be, I am not a balanced meal."

"Wow, you are amazing! Our Grandpa needs your help for his heart problems," Sax says in awe.

Mrs. Strawberry, looking fondly at them, answers, "I'm always happy to make new friends. Good luck with your mission, children."

"Thanks for everything!" Sammie and Sax say together as Sax drags Rhubarb away from the baby strawberries.

Raising his nose and sniffing the air, Rhubarb charges into the deep woods.

"After him!" Sammie shouts, and the children race through the trees.

"WROOF, WROOF!"

"SQUAAWWK!"

"WROOF! WROOF!"

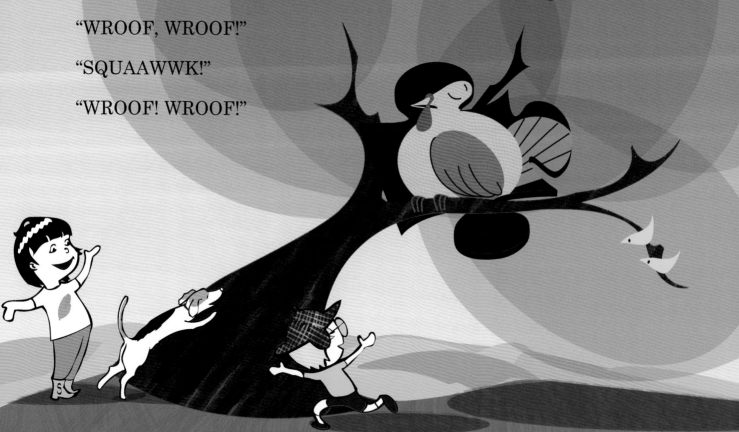

"SQUAAAAWK! Well, I never! Disturbing my sleep like that!" a great big turkey declares, ruffling his feathers.

"Rhubarb, please stop barking! It's just a turkey!" Sax pleads.

"Just a turkey? I am not JUST a turkey, young boy," Mr. Turkey gobbles.

"If you must know, my meat is most people's favorite and makes your muscles strong; it also gives you more energy to play and think … which I see you need!"

"Sorry to disturb you, sir. So does this mean you're the balanced meal we've been looking for? We're on a mission, you see," Sammie explains.

"Grumpf," Mr. Turkey grumbles, "I'm afraid you and your dog are barking up the wrong tree. Even with my leading role in your Thanksgiving dinner, I alone am not a balanced meal. On you go with your mission. Wander into town and ask someone else. SQUAWWK! I need to finish my nap. And take that noisy dog with you!"

Sax answers with a sigh, "Okay. Thanks for your help. We'll be going now. C'mon Rhubarb, c'mon Sammie. Let's walk back to the road."

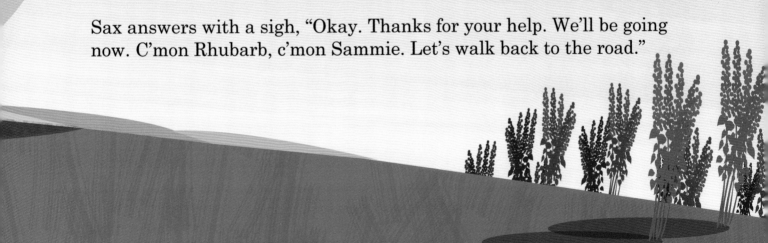

"Hello, children. I am Miss Catherine BeMine Cake. You look lost and a bit hungry. Can I help you? How about some teacakes and milk? And here's a saucer to give your dog some water."

Sammie stands tall and says, "We are not lost, Miss BeMine Cake. We're on a mission to find a balanced meal!"

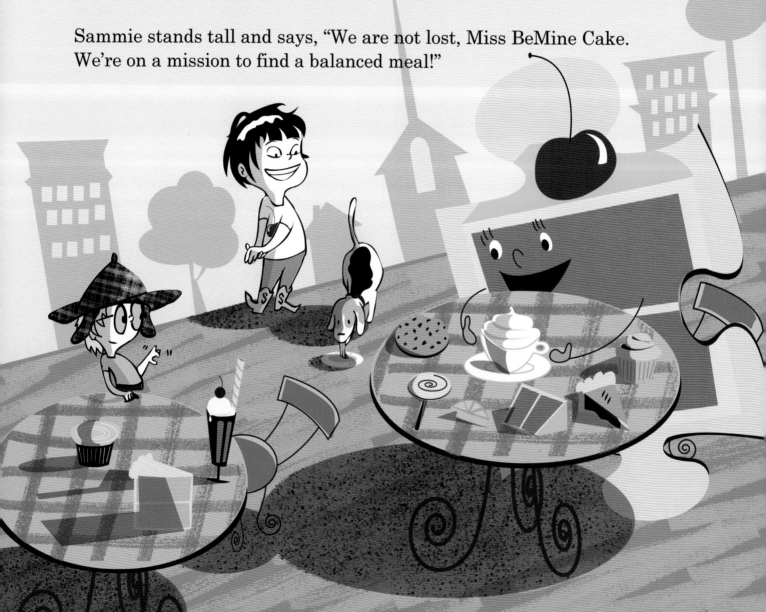

"Oooh! How exciting! You must be starving! How about a bite of my frosting? It's cherry-chocolate-caramel-marshmallow cream," Miss BeMine Cake says temptingly.

"This looks so amazing! Are you perhaps a balanced meal?" Sax gasps. "I sure hope so!"

"Well, I'm quite BEE-YOU-TEE-FULL and so SWEET, but I haven't a clue what you mean by a balanced meal. It sounds serious and no one takes me seriously, dear ones. I'm just for fun. People love to invite me to parties, but I'm not much help. Go talk to someone at the Farmers' Market. I'm sure they'll help," she says with a sweet grin. "Take a few cookies with you. Don't eat them all! They're good for getting people talking."

With a noisy smack of his lips, Sax responds, "All right, Miss BeMine Cake."

"Thanks for the cookies," Sammie adds as they walk on.

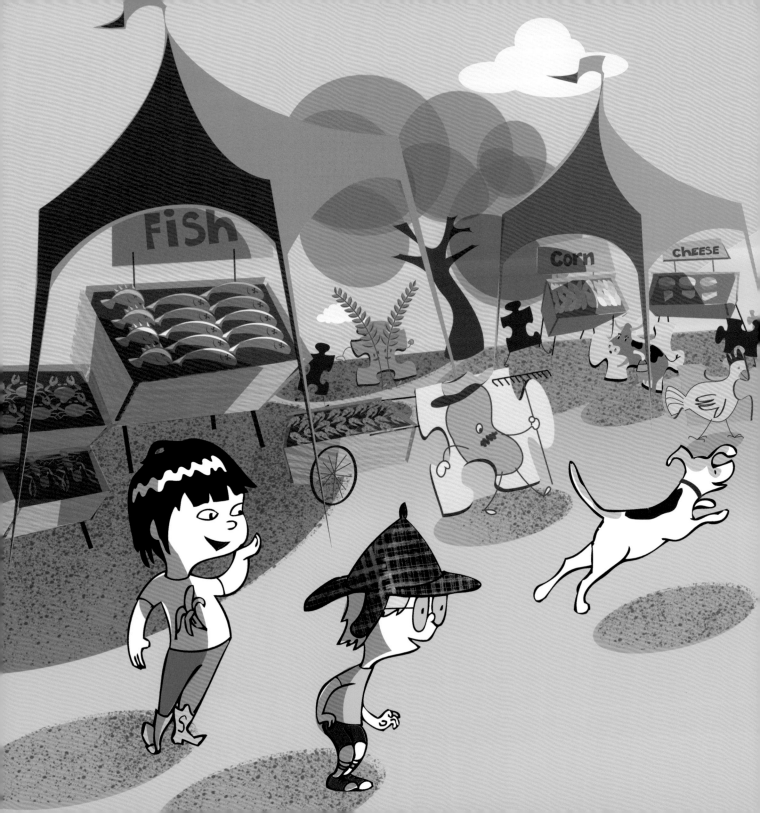

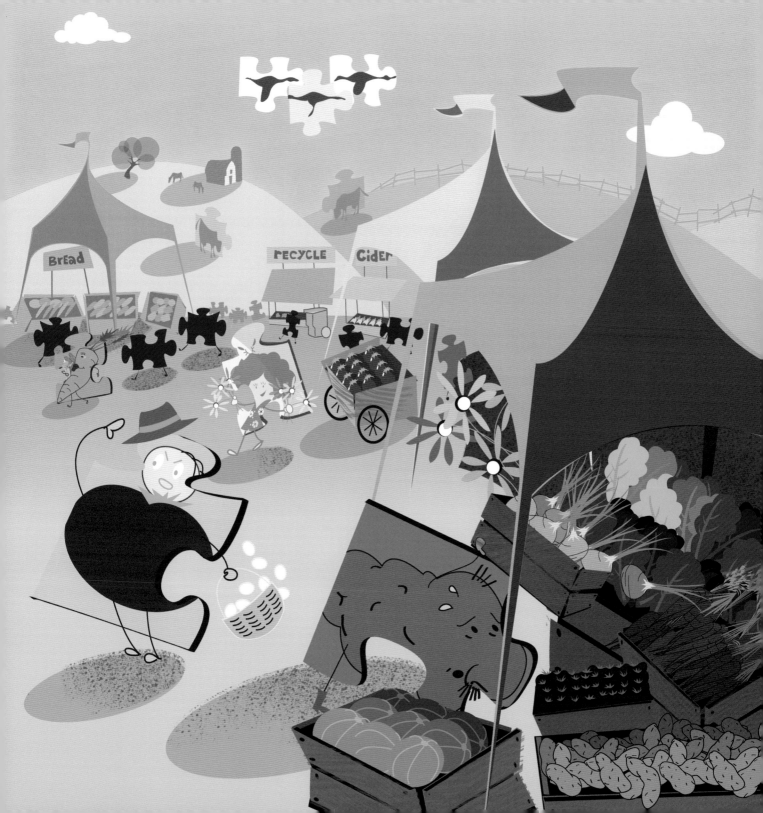

After walking around the Farmers' Market for a while, Sammie decides to visit Mr. Sweet Potato at his vegetable stand. "Hello, sir. We are wondering if you can help us?"

"Too busy, children. Too busy!" Mr. Sweet Potato says, hurriedly.

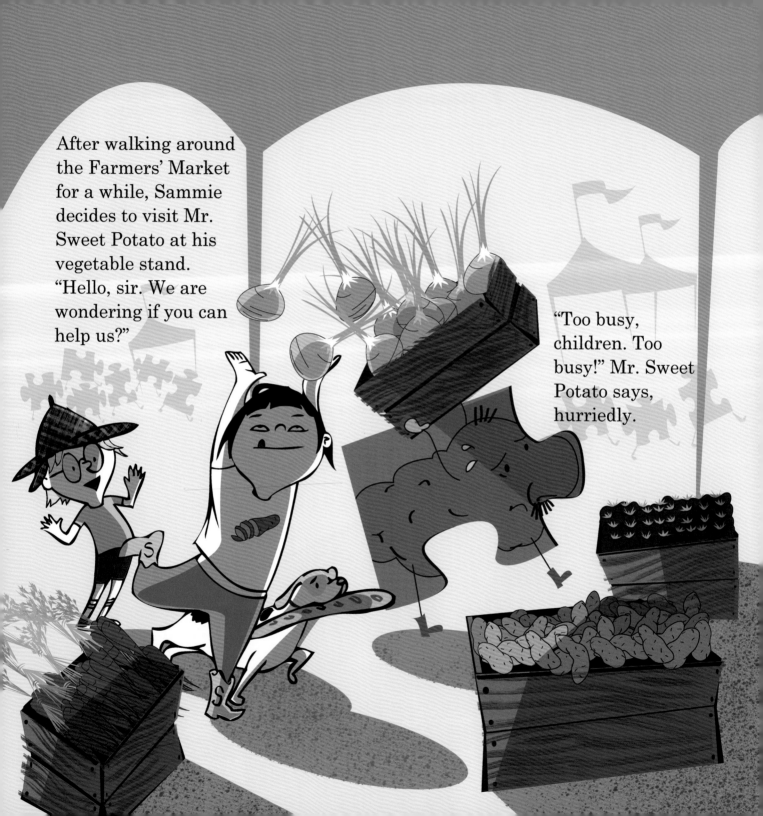

"If you tell us you're a balanced meal, we have a cookie from Miss BeMine Cake for you." Sax smiles, hopefully.

Mr. Sweet Potato pauses and grins, "Are you trying to sweet talk a sweet potato? Well, for your information I'm also a hearty food that protects people from nasty colds and builds strong bones. But sadly, I am not your answer to a balanced meal."

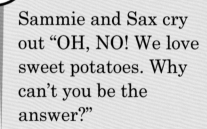

Sammie and Sax cry out "OH, NO! We love sweet potatoes. Why can't you be the answer?"

"I am so tired. My curiosity cap is all thought out!
We have talked to so many foods, and they have all given us
the same answer," Sax groans, leaning against Rhubarb.
In a sad, small voice he adds,
"It looks like there is not any **ONE** food
that makes a balanced meal!"

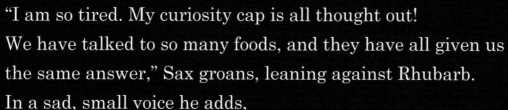

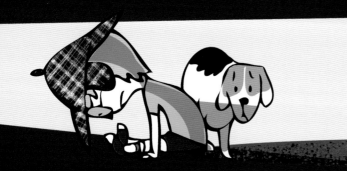

Sammie pouts,
"Looks like we will **NEVER** find an answer
on this adventure."

"What will we tell Mama? What will
we eat for dinner? We can't go back now!
Somebody has to help us!" Sax pleads,
looking around the Farmers' Market.

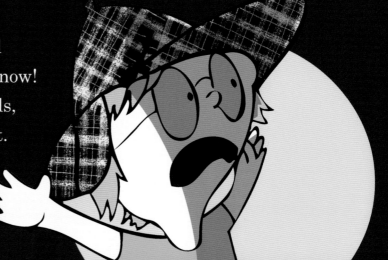

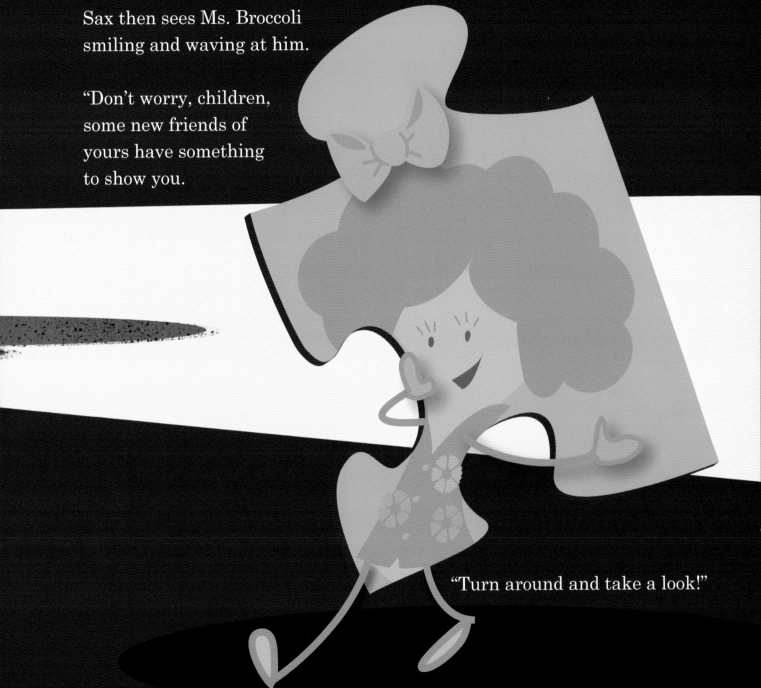

Sax then sees Ms. Broccoli smiling and waving at him.

"Don't worry, children, some new friends of yours have something to show you.

"Turn around and take a look!"

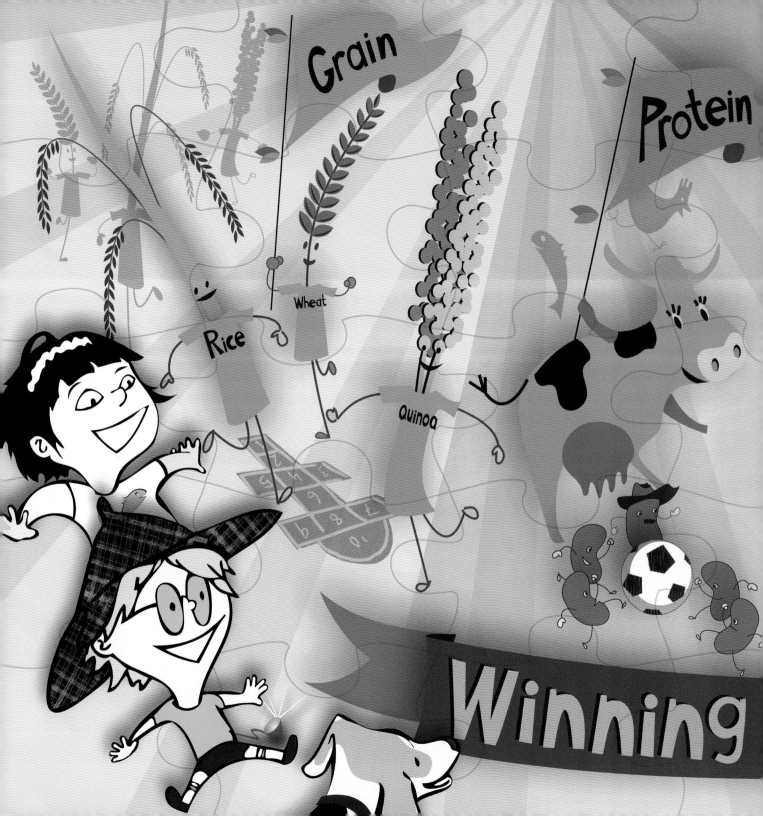

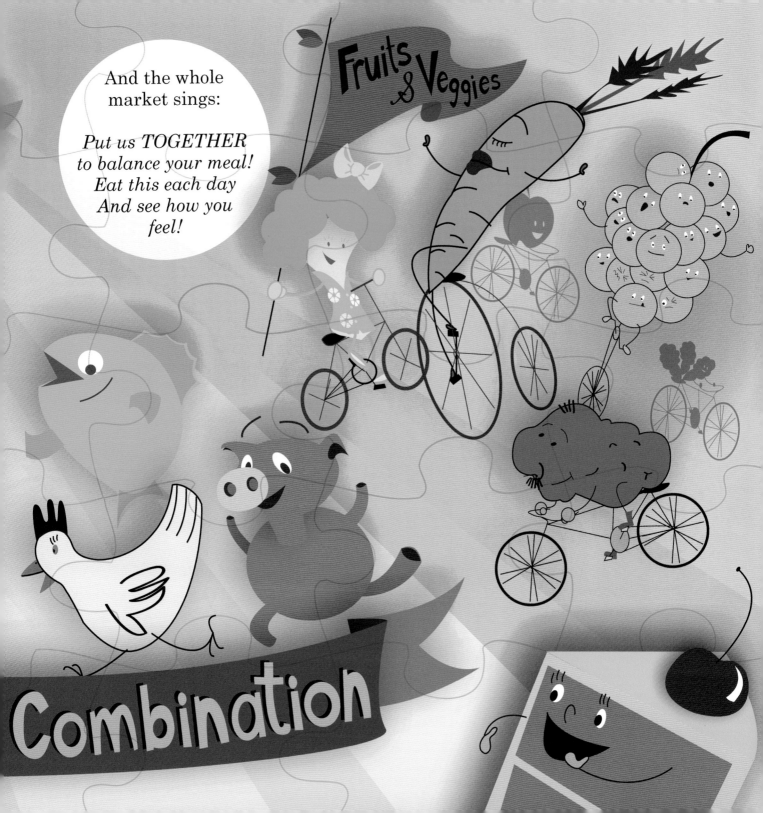

"So that's why you're all puzzle-piece-food people!"
Sammie says happily.
"You fit together to keep us healthy!"

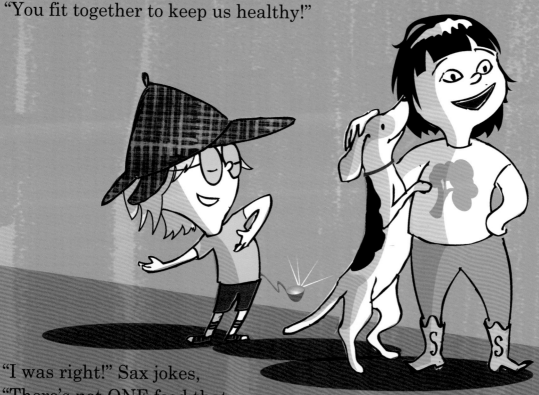

"I was right!" Sax jokes,
"There's not ONE food that
makes a balanced meal! We need vegetables like broccoli, fruits
like berries, meats like turkey, and carbs like sweet potatoes or
grains like quinoa! That's what balanced means! A meal with
ALL of these foods!"

"Now we can go home and plan our own balanced meal!"
Sammie claps her hands with joy, "Sax! Prepare to *ZOOM*!"

"Ready?" Sammie asks.

"Ready!" Sax replies.

Sammie begins her
Spoon Zoom rhyme:

Oh, balanced meals
Are you big, are you lean?
Are you French Fries on wheels?
Are you towers of beans?

Back home we zoom!
With our dinner to make
Oh, magical spoon
You helped balance our plate!

And together the children shout,
"SPOON ZOOM, AWAY!"

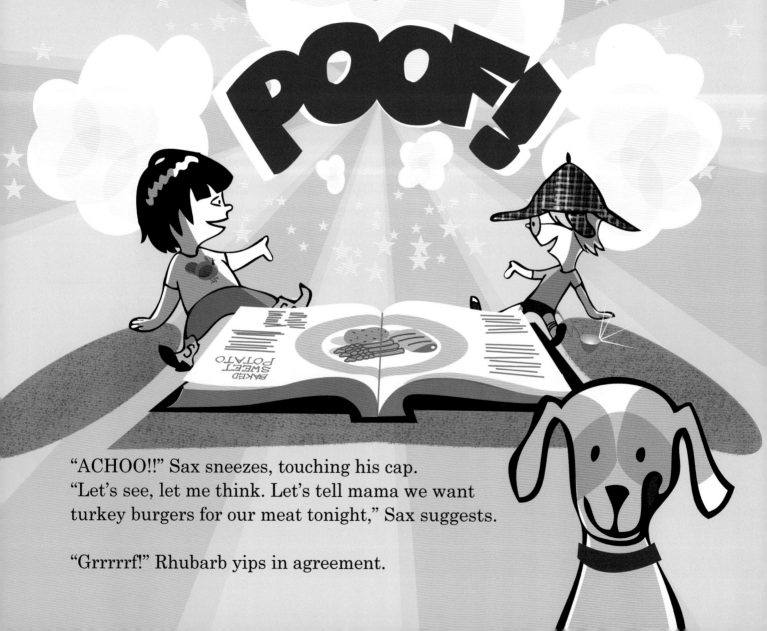

Sitting back by the cookbook, Sammie says, "Balanced meals are awesome! Just like fitting pieces of a puzzle together. And with so many different choices, it never gets boring!"

"ACHOO!!" Sax sneezes, touching his cap. "Let's see, let me think. Let's tell mama we want turkey burgers for our meat tonight," Sax suggests.

"Grrrrrf!" Rhubarb yips in agreement.

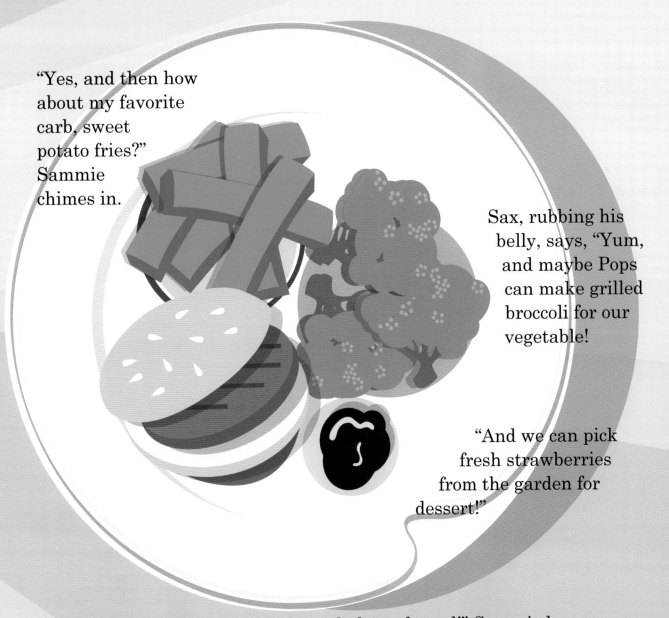

"Yes, and then how about my favorite carb, sweet potato fries?" Sammie chimes in.

Sax, rubbing his belly, says, "Yum, and maybe Pops can make grilled broccoli for our vegetable!

"And we can pick fresh strawberries from the garden for dessert!"

"Looks like we have put together a balanced meal!" Sammie beams. "Mission accomplished!" Sax agrees as Rhubarb licks his face.

"SHHLURP!"

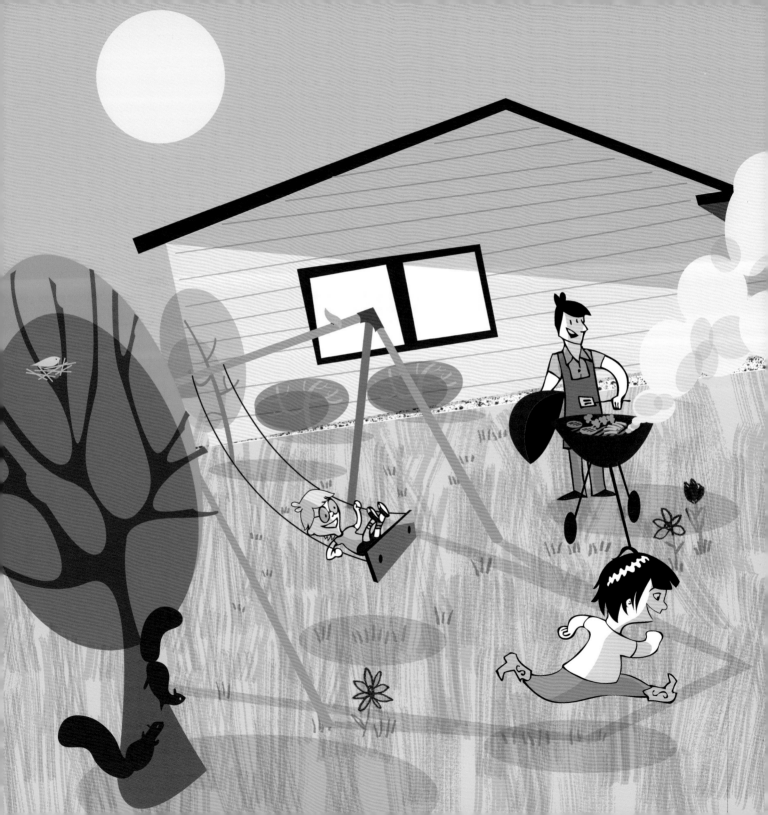

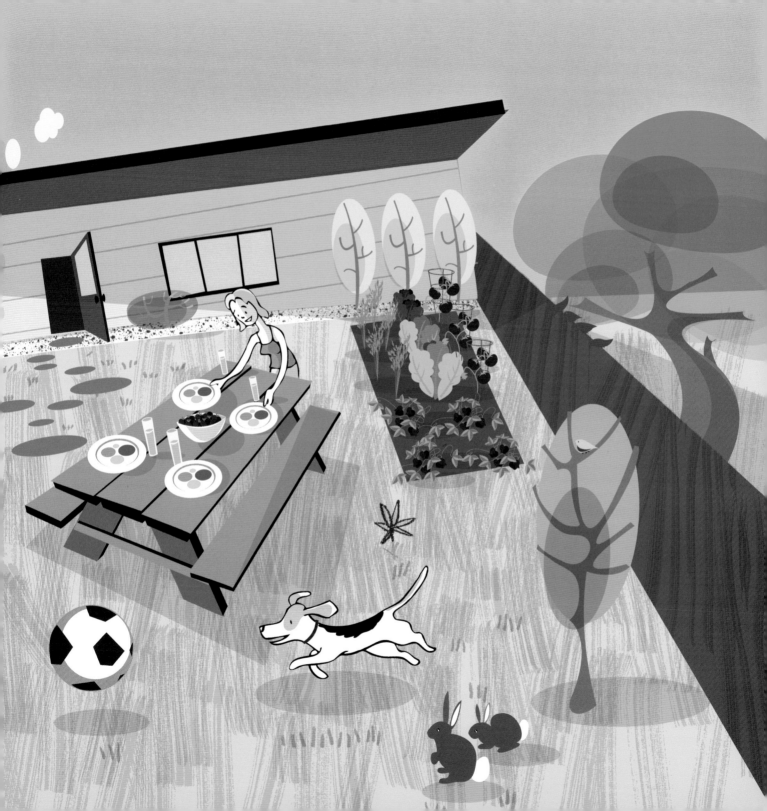

Recipes

Farmers' Market Turkey Burger

1 lb. ground turkey
½ cup whole wheat Panko breadcrumbs
¼ cup onion, finely chopped
1 garlic clove, minced
2 Tbsp. parsley, finely chopped
⅛ cup ketchup
¼ tsp. black pepper
½ tsp. oregano
2 egg whites, lightly beaten
non-stick cooking spray
4 slices cheese, cheddar, 2% milk
4 slices tomato
4 whole wheat buns

Instructions:

1. Combine first 8 ingredients in a bowl; add egg whites and mix until well blended.
2. Divide mixture into 4 equal parts, shape each into a ½ inch thick patty.
3. Coat a medium nonstick skillet with cooking spray, place over medium heat until hot.
4. Add patties, cook 5 to 6 minutes on each side or until done.
5. Place a cheese slice on each patty while still in skillet.
6. Serve patties on buns and top with tomato.

Serve hot
Serves 4; Calories 380 per serving

Wild Sweet Potato Fries

2 medium sweet potatoes, scrubbed
salt, pepper
1 Tbsp. herbes de Provence
¾ tsp. garlic powder, California style
non-stick cooking spray, olive oil flavored

Instructions:

1. Preheat oven to 400°F.
2. Spray baking sheet with cooking spray.
3. Slice the potatoes lengthwise into ¼-inch thick slices. Then cut again to make fries to your preferred size.
4. Place them in a large bowl and spray them with cooking spray; sprinkle them with the herbes de Provence, garlic powder, ground pepper and salt. Toss to coat.
5. Arrange potatoes on the baking sheet.
6. Bake fries until golden and tender, about 35 – 45 minutes.

Serve hot
Serves 4; Calories 77 per serving

Mission Accomplished Grilled Broccoli

1 broccoli bunch, cut into 8 large spears
2 lemons, quartered
1 tsp. garlic powder, California style
1 tsp. olive oil
¼ tsp. kosher salt
¼ tsp. pepper, (coarse ground)
non-stick cooking spray, olive oil flavored

Instructions:

1. Heat grill to medium.
2. In a medium bowl, toss broccoli with lemons, oil and spices.
3. Spray grill with non-stick cooking spray.
4. Grill broccoli and lemon, turning occasionally until tender and lightly charred, 10 – 15 minutes.

Serve hot
Serves 4; Calories 42 per serving

From the Patch Fresh Strawberries

1 Quart Strawberries

Instructions:

1. Wash strawberries, leaving the stems on.
2. Divide the strawberries into 4 equal portions, and place them in 4 bowls.

Serves 4; Calories 24 per serving

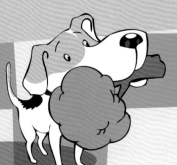

For more recipes go to our website
www.livligahome.com

Balanced Meal Lesson & Learning

Balanced Meal Lesson:

We need to supply our body with the nourishment it needs so our brains can think, our eyes can see, our muscles can move, our bones stay strong, and so we have the energy to do the things we need and want to do. By eating a balanced meal, which includes a variety of foods, our body gets what it needs to do its job. If we exclude important food groups and the nourishment they provide, our body cannot do its job.

Lesson Learned:

A balanced meal is made up of many different foods. They fit together like pieces of a puzzle. You just need to figure out which puzzle pieces to include in order to make each meal a balanced meal. You do this by choosing one food item from each food group.

Conversation Questions:

1.   What food groups need to be included for a balanced meal?
2.   Which foods give you energy?
3.   Why is it important to combine foods?
4.   Does a cupcake make a balanced meal?
5.   On your plate, you have chicken, quinoa, and some mustard. What needs to be added to make a balanced meal: mac and cheese, snap peas, or a brownie?

About the Author

Sheila is first and foremost the mom of three children. They have been her inspiration and source of passion for many of the endeavors she has pursued over the years. Sheila is also a storyteller. When her kids were little she would tell them *Kingdom of Good* stories at bedtime. These stories would take them to a magical land where they discovered many things, learned about challenges and how they had the solutions within themselves to solve the problems at hand. This new series of books, starting with *Sammie & Sax in the Land of Quinoa,* has been inspired by those original stories.

Sheila is the Founder and CEO of Livliga—a brand of healthy, artist-designed dinnerware products to help people and families live healthier lives. Before launching her own company she was the Executive Director of the American Heart Association in Denver. Early on, after college, Sheila was also a teacher in a small village in Zaïre called Kasando as a Peace Corps volunteer. She currently lives in Boulder, Colorado, with her husband, Walt, to whom she has been married for thirty years.

About the Illustrator

As a kid, Timothy Foss preferred art supply stores over toy stores, and could spend hours choosing a pencil. He grew up, attended St. Olaf College, discovered his love for ceramics, and moved to Seattle to begin a decade-long career that culminated in a series he called *Poor Man's Porcelain.* Examples of this work can be found in the collections of the San Francisco Museum of Fine Art-Deyoung, Arizona State University, and the Museum of Contemporary Craft-Portland.

He received an MFA at the University of Colorado, and realized that storytelling guided all of his work. Now he feels right at home as the Chief Creative Officer for Livliga—designing ceramics and building the visual story of Sammie and Sax. His 3-year-old son, Eli, has tested all of the contents of this book (he approves). You can find his family in Minneapolis curled up on a chair somewhere reading books.

About Livliga

To find out more about Livliga, visit our website at www.livligahome.com. You can also visit the Livliga blog through our website, or follow Livliga at facebook.com/livligahome, twitter.com/livligahome and pinterest.com/livligahome.